The 21 Indispensable Qualities of a Nurse

Eva M Francis, MSN, RN, CCRN

ACKNOWLEDGEMENTS

This book is dedicated to all nurses across the globe who have dedicated their lives and time to serve mankind.

As Nurses we believe that patients and families are the most important in the healthcare equation and our goal is to serve with passion, power, patience and pride.

Table of Contents

Introduction: The 21 Characteristics of a GREAT NURSE

Do you know that at the time of this writing Nurses were voted the most trusted professionals BY THE Gallup Poll for over 16 years in the arrow? Nurses have been proven and seen as the heart and soul of health care. They are the heroes of today and the heroes of tomorrow. I firmly believe that the power of nursing is a definite calling. One cannot survive or function in nursing without the mindset that its all about people. Once that is engraved in the mind of a nurse, then everything else will fall into place.

The Great John C Maxwell says, "Leadership is an influence, nothing more and nothing less. I want to describe Nursing as Caring and Compassion. Nothing more and nothing less! Everything that we embrace as a Nurse is in alignment with Care and Compassion.

The Nursing profession is widely recognized as one of the most interpersonal careers in the world, whereby close relationships are established between nurse practitioners and their patients. For this sole reason, it is undisputed that nurses make a profound difference in the lives of the patients who regard their services as indispensable. Having acquired knowledge through their years in Nursing school, nurses apply what they have learned to ensure quality patient care. By contributing significantly to patients' mental and physical wellbeing, nurses inherently become pioneers of the success and stability of health care institutions. Nevertheless, individuals who succeed in nursing and gain fulfillment in their career must possess unique qualities such as caring, compassion, confidence, commitment, community, consistency, communication skills, competence, courage, capability, and connectedness.

Furthermore, one must understand that before success comes leadership. Put, leadership entails a multifaceted approach whereby one person serves as a guide for a group of people who assemble to reach a common goal or objective. For effective and successful leadership, the unique qualities mentioned above—communication, commitment, courage, etc.—stand as the pillars of a strong foundation upon which a leader provides a change in their community, be it the healthcare institution or otherwise. Hence, it is essential to note that success and leadership are not mutually exclusive as the specific impact measures success and legacy leaders leave for those around them.

This book, "The 21 C's for Great Leadership," serves as a manual that outlines the 21 unique and essential qualities required for every individual to invest in their self-development to be the best and most successful version of oneself. As this book progresses, you will see the intersection of all 21 qualities to be discussed. It will serve as a reminder that the effort you put into yourself and others cannot be made halfway—what is worth doing is worth doing well.

Chapter 1
Caring

"Friendly people are caring people, eager to provide encouragement and support when needed most" – Rosabeth Moss Kanter

No one can ever underestimate the fact that as nurses caring is our life. Our patients are at our mercy and we have no choice but to give them our all when they show up in our organizations . No matter if we are direct caregiver or indirect caregiver, we are essentially servants leaders to those we are called to serve.

I remember many years ago, I took care of a patient in the Critical Care Unit as an ICU Nurse, with a very distraught family who was extremely angry and sad about their loved one. I remember as a brand new ICU Nurse, I took the time to meet with the family to give them some update about the patient. One thing I remember telling her is that we have seen sicker patients walk out of this hospital. Somehow they held on to that little glimmer of hope. The patient eventually went home .

After twenty years, I was attendfing a wedding in another state and saw a couple running to hug me, they reminded me that I took care of their son twenty years prior. I vaguely remember the patient, however they clearly remembered all the details.

The morale of this story is this: Every moment with these patients matters. They should never be taken for granted. Patients will share some sensitive secrets with us that they will never even share with another family member. The trust that is placed upon us is a huge responsibility and in the caring characteristic, they hold on to our trust.

Caring is the heart of the nursing profession. Nurses demonstrate caring by focusing not only on the physical, but also the mind and the spirit of the patients. Therefore, great nurses must view the patient as a whole by recognizing the interdependence between their physical, psychological, and spiritual well-being. Caring nurses should incorporate a wide range of approaches when meeting the needs of the patients, including the delivery of the appropriate medication, education, communication, and complementary treatment. Moreover, caring nurses must consider all the aspects of the patients' treatment by considering their thoughts, emotions, culture, opinions, and attitudes because they play a significant role in the healing process and improves patient satisfaction.

Caring enables nurses to respect patients' dignity. Through caring, the relationship between the nurses and the patients is based on respect and mutuality because patients are allowed to participate in decision making. The nurses delivering holistic care, respect the patient's role in the treatment process. The aspect of respecting the patient's concerns enables nurses to better understand the effects of an illness on the patient's life. As a result, they encourage the patients to take part in the treatment process by providing education and encouraging them to embrace self-care. Self-care enables the patients to perform their daily activities independently, improves the quality of the patients' life, and self-confidence. Consequently, caring nurses are great because they encourage self-discipline, vigor, and a sense of autonomy. In so doing, caring heals the whole of a person by improving the harmony between the patient's body, mind, and spirit.

According to James Keller, "a candle loses nothing by lighting another candle." As nurses and individuals at large, caring for others is a paramount quality for exceptional leadership. Showing concern for the well being of others is an indication of selfless leadership and motivation to ensure the best for those placed under your responsibility, and not yourself alone. If one shows no care, there is no will to make an impact—inherently leaving that individual in a state of stagnation. We can only rise by lifting others.

Chapter 2
Compassionate

"There is a nobility in compassion, a beauty in empathy, a grace in forgiveness." – John Connolly

Compassion refers to how care is given to patients through relationships that are based on dignity. The study further argues that empathy is also described as acts of kindness. Compassion is essential in nursing because it determines how the patients perceive their care. Today, nurses must be compassionate due to the ever-increasing impersonal technology that has been adopted in health care. The advantages of technology in healthcare cannot be overlooked. They include effective communication, the efficiency of care, and improved patient safety. However, the overreliance on technology has adversely affected the nurse's behavior as well as the nurse-patient relationship. Some nurse solely relies on the information provided by the technological systems and fail to consider and respect the personal information provided by the patient. As a result, relationship-based care is neglected.

The nurses must be compassionate and resist the technological dehumanization, which encourages them to overshadow the personhood of the recipients of care. The nurse must learn to use technology as a tool to improve their ability to deliver care to the patients. Although the technology in the health facilities is louder than the patients, the nurse must learn to pay attention to the patient's stories, experiences, and concerns rather than the technological devices. Over reliance on healthcare technology to make informed decisions about the patients' problems jeopardizes the nurses' opportunity to be with and know the patients. Consequently, nursing activities such as touch, attentiveness, listening, and presence should be prioritized. These aspects enable nurses to recognize the patient's suffering and to take the necessary actions to relieve the pain.

As a leader, regardless of the position, you are put in or the pedestal you have been placed on, remember that those around you—whether they are your employees, coworkers, colleagues—are human beings like you before anything else. With compassion comes humility, and one must be able to understand that no condition is permanent— being the boss today doesn't guarantee that you will be the boss forever. This is why being humble and having a sense of humanity goes hand in hand towards formulating a compassionate individual and an effective leader.

Chapter 3
Confidence

"Confidence comes not from always being right but from not fearing to be wrong" -Peter T. Mcintyre

Confidence is a characteristic of caring in nursing that binds various C's together. Individuals must have confidence in the nursing skills and knowledge to be committed in the delivery of quality care, to consistently act courageously and competently, and to express compassion and care, even in complex situations. Nurses must be confident to deliver quality care to the patients effectively. Confidence is the individual's freedom from doubting his/her beliefs and abilities. In nursing, professional confidence is associated with the delivery of care to the patients. Trust is essential in nursing because self-doubt interferes with their ability to acquire new knowledge and limits their ability to tackle difficult situations. The idea of instilling confidence in the nurses provides the foundation for successful implementation and acquisition of new skills. Belief is the foundation for the nurses' motivation, wellbeing, and personal accomplishment.

In nursing, it takes time to become familiar with new responsibilities. However, the stakes are high because one small mistake can result in the patient's death. The pressure when managing a new role can lead the nurses to chronic distress and self-doubt. Confidence issues are not only limited to new and inexperienced nurses; sometimes, even the skilled nurses experience challenges they have never dealt with before. Therefore, since nurses cannot fake skills and knowledge that they do not have, they need confidence. Confidence improves the nurses' ability to leverage the resources they have and enhance patient care instead of focusing on the knowledge gap. A confident nurse is great because she invokes positive change in the patient's care and improves their quality of life.

Moreover, confidence and conceitedness are often misconstrued in leadership. The former refers to one's appreciation of their abilities and the impact it can make, while the latter begs a vain, individualistic, and self-centered approach to leadership. Distinguishing between both is very crucial because the failure of most leaders occurs when their confidence develops into conceitedness. There is nothing wrong with being aware of one's talents and abilities. Still, the moment one expresses self-appreciation to bring others down or to feel they are 'above,' the results can be catastrophic. Understanding that your strengths may be the weaknesses of others (and vice versa) will enable you to apply your confidence in a collaborative way whereby others can learn from you while simultaneously, you can learn from them.

Confidence comes with believing in oneself. It is said that when we believe in ourself, we can chart the course of our path with confidence.

Chapter 4
Commitment

"Motivation is what gets you started. Commitment is what keeps you going." - Jim Rohn

Commitment to the populations and individual patients is the cornerstone of the nursing practice; this is because it is the obligation to deliver quality care. Strong commitment enables the nurses to believe in their patients' values and autonomy. Great nurses build on their promise by holistically examining the experience of each patient and sourcing for different methods to facilitate patient recovery and development. For example, nurses who promptly respond to the patient's concerns are dedicated to providing optimal care that improves the patient's well being and overall satisfaction.

Nursing theorists such as Florence Nightingale emphasize the commitment to nursing work. The researcher argues that caring behaviors with commitment include attending to the patients regardless of the critical situation such as the dying process and times. Nightingale encourages the nurses to be committed to sustaining care and compassionate relationships in healthcare and the development of self and others. The highly committed nurses are responsible for delivering high-quality care to the patients. Further, they maintain their commitment by keeping the pledge and being honest when performing their obligations to the healthcare profession and the patients. The engagement enhances patient safety and the wellbeing of the patients. Further, the nurses who demonstrate commitment also to stay in their work for a more extended period, thus minimizing high turnover rates and absenteeism, which adversely affect the quality of care delivered to the patients. Consequently, a strong commitment to nursing has essential consequences in healthcare because it contributes to the success of health care institutions.

Chapter 5
Community

"The greatness of a community is most accurately measured by the compassionate actions of its members." – Coretta Scott King.

A community in nursing is indicative of the long and short-term provision of care to individuals and their families to enhance their capacity for self-care. The population in nursing is a fundamental entity that encourages the nurses not to focus on the health of one patient at a time, but the community as a whole. Further, community-based nursing provides that the patients survive within a culture, community, family, and society. Therefore, the nurses must understand all these interactions when delivering care to the patients. The care takes place in the clinic as well as homes. The nurses should develop community practice proficiency to advance the quality of care they deliver to the patient in small communities, rural, and urban areas. The community practice is based on critical thinking when assessing health status, identifying the appropriate nursing interventions, and evaluating the outcomes of the care delivered.

The nurses should develop community practice proficiency because many challenges have adverse effects on the patients in the community. They include infectious diseases such as tuberculosis, preventable diseases such as injuries, obesity, and environmental toxins. These factors, among others, increase morbidity and mortality among pregnant women, infants, and other vulnerable populations. Community practice proficiency entails awareness on significant and minor community health issues and requires nurses to apply their knowledge towards improving the health outcomes of these populations. Some of the activities that should be conducted by nurses include assessment, vaccination, and screening. The interventions are essential because the nurses are encouraged to promote prevention over treatment in the community. When they correct poor health practices, they lower the patient's risk and reduce the number of visits to the healthcare facilities.

Considering those as mentioned above, it is crucial to understand that a nurse should educate members of their community about prevalent health issues they face, the causes of these issues, and preventative measures that members of the community can come together to execute. Exhibiting such an approach often leads to drastic declines in epidemics of, i.e., Malaria, Cholera, when awareness is created with the use of, i.e., mosquito nets, etc.

We have a great responsibility to our community to serve. As I always say, we are on stage as nurses and our community is looking to us for guidance.

Our community needs us.

Chapter 6
Consistent

"Success isn't always about greatness. It's about consistency. Consistent hard work leads to success. Greatness will come." - Dwayne Johnson

Great nurses must be consistent in regards to patience supervision. Consistency focuses on the regularity of quality care provided. It is also important to note that consistency is the vital pathway required for all individuals to reach success. Consistency in interventions is essential due to the ongoing changes in health care delivery. In the absence of compatibility, nurses can quickly lose sight of the immutable facts in their practice. Meeting the needs of patients from different backgrounds requires a comprehensive care plan. To meet the changes in health care, the care plan can be monitored by clinical professionals when necessary. Healthcare plans are indispensable resources that effectively guide the nurse's practice. Additionally, consistency is essential when developing a care plan because it standardizes the nurse's practices and encourages them to use evidence-based practices to improve the quality of care delivered to the patients and their wellbeing.

Furthermore, consistency in nursing aids is the proper prevention of medical errors. At least one-third of errors occur during the nurse administration phase. These mistakes result in adverse events, consequently compromising the patient's safety. Errors result in unwarranted financial burdens needed to alleviate the consequences of a practitioner's miscalculation. Hence, to avoid such mishaps, a successful nurse must pair consistency with CAUTION—that is, standard healthcare procedures must be accorded with attentiveness and alertness. Therefore, the nurses must be consistent because the administration of the medication to the patients tend to be very risky.

Moreover, consistent advocates for the continuity of care over a patient. The nurse does not forget about the patient once they have been discharged from the clinic. This is one of the avenues where successful nurses intersect commitment, care, and consistency by monitoring the patient's progress even when they leave the hospital. Following up after treatment entails observing the patient's improvement to ensure that their health status is up to par, and this yields a marked advancement in their quality of life.

Put, consistency, and caution promote a safe and productive environment in healthcare institutions, while simultaneously improving long-lasting interpersonal relationships between nurse practitioners and their patients.

Chapter 7
Communication

Communication - the human connection - is the key to personal and career success. - Paul J. Meyer

Communication in healthcare is paramount and is one of the most effective tool we have for providing great patient care as well as patient satisfaction improvement.

Communication is a universal foundation of relationships between individuals all around the world. It is the blueprint upon which awareness is created and the clay from which formulas for change are molded. Communication is the core of successful, caring relationships in nursing practice. Effective communication encourages nurses to develop effective teamwork, which improves the wellbeing of the patient. Communication is integral to the values of other C's, such as caring, compassion, and competence. Excellent communication makes nurses great because all the interventions, including prevention, treatment, rehabilitation, education, and health promotion, are enhanced through interpersonal communication. Through an interface, the nurses can exchange information, thoughts, and feelings with the patients and their families. Further, communication is a two-way process. Therefore, the patients also share their concerns and fears with the nurses. Nurses must be good listeners. By listening, they can assess the patient's problems, enhance the individual's self-esteem, and integrate nursing diagnosis. Effective communication enables nurses to correct the diagnosis.

Further, understanding the patients' concerns is central to the delivery of patient-centered care. The nurses should have a sincere intention to understand the patient's interest. To understand the patient's fears and concerns, the nurse must convey their messages in an understandable and acceptable language. The nurses should not use technical terms and medical terminologies when communicating with the patients, when the patients cannot understand the technical jargon used by the patients, their developmental stress, thus making it difficult for the nurse and the patient to communicate. Nonverbal communication is also vital in health care. The nurses should pay attention to facial expressions, gestures, and the patient's posture. These elements are essential for patients to feel comfortable when communicating with nurses.

Chapter 8
Competence

"Success demands a high level of logistical and organizational competence." – George S. Patton

According to the Health Stream, competence is the "application and demonstration of appropriate knowledge, skills, behaviors, and judgment in a clinical setting." Fitness is measured by the accuracy and effectiveness in which learned skills are put into practice to achieve consistent results.

Competent nurses must have the capability to care and recognize the patient's health and social needs. They should also have the expertise, clinical, and technical knowledge that will enable them to deliver efficient care and treatment according to evidence-based research. Competent nurses are skilled and consistent in their performance. Great nurses must be qualified because healthcare has changed due to factors such as the rapidly aging population and the changes in disease structure. Healthcare systems have also changed. For example, when an individual is presented to the hospital with an acute illness, the nurses are expected to provide short term and intensive care. Upon the completion of the treatment, home care is recommended to ensure that the patient is treated with dignity and respect until the end of their life. Regardless of the setting, only competent nurses can deliver comprehensive care that meets the patient's complex and diverse health care needs.

Competence is essential in nursing because it enables nurses to perform their core duties. Nursing competence is an integration of professional skills, values, and attitudes. The nurses are required to utilize nursing knowledge and nursing judgment when assessing the health needs of the patients and providing care and advice to support the patients to manage their health. Competence in nursing also relates to the legal and ethical responsibility of the nurses. Great nurses require proficiency to demonstrate knowledge and to be accountable for their actions and decisions. Competence further enables the nurses to develop therapeutic and interpersonal communication with the patients and nursing staff. Accordingly, they maximize patient safety, independence, and quality of life.

Chapter 9
Courageous

"Success is not final, and failure is not fatal: it is the courage to continue that counts." – Winston S. Churchill

When reflecting on this final project, courage was perhaps one of the most controversial and practical "C" that was identified. The reason being, in most cases, when asked to identify a caring profession, nursing comes to mind. However, when individuals are asked to identify a courageous declaration, they define jobs such as firefighting, police work, and entrepreneurship. It is miserable because nursing is overlooked, yet, in reality, the nurses cannot deliver quality care without being courageous. Courage is a fundamental virtue of nursing success. For example, it takes courage to comfort a sick or dying person, to question the physician's recommendations, and respect the patient's concerns regardless of their cultural beliefs and gender.

Great nurses must be courageous because they are exposed to various challenges in their practice. The most common problems include overburdened workloads, managing change in healthcare, and confronting fear. Nurses must be courageous to facilitate sustainable change in health care. They must face their fears and engage the principles that support quality care for the patients. Courage also enables the nurse to manage moral distress, including the conflicts that arise when the nurses' commitment to an organization is misaligned with their duty to the patients. When the battle continues over a long period, nurses develop chronic stress, burnout, and lack of focus. Courage is, therefore, an essential component because it enables the nurses to resolve the distress. They can do the right thing for the patients and to speak up when they have concerns. Courage in nursing can be developed through education and training. Knowledge enables the nurses to build personal strength and to do what is right in the event of inevitable obstacles and barriers.

Chapter 10
Capable

"We are all strangers to our hidden potential until we confront problems that reveal our capabilities" – Nathaniel Branden

Capability in nursing is a fundamental aspect that makes nurses great due to the volatile nature of the healthcare industry. Today, technology, information, and science are within the public's reach. As a result, the professions, particularly nursing, are confronted with the need to improve their quality of work and processes to advance the well being of the patients and their quality of life. The nurses must be capable because the advances in healthcare technology have increased costs in the healthcare sector as well as the population's expectations concerning the quality of services delivered. Despite the changes in the healthcare industry, when the nurses are capable, they improve efficiency and efficacy and minimize the flaws in the quality and safety of care.

Successful nurses are aware of their responsibility to take into account the patient's expectations in decision making. In so doing, patient satisfaction is improved. Patient satisfaction is essential because it has been identified as a care quality indicator. The reason being, listening to what the recipients of care say about the care they receive is an excellent opportunity to construct an outcome indicator, which provides an opportunity for the nurse leaders to decide on the transformation required in the healthcare facility. The experience of the patients serves as an indicator for evaluating and improving the quality of care delivered by the nurses. When the nurse leaders assess the patient's skills, they use the results for internal quality improvement. Nurses can use patient expectations and experiences to adjust their practice and to improve patient outcomes.

Chapter 11
Connectedness

"Whatever affects one directly, affects all indirectly. I can never be what I ought to be until you are what you ought to be" – Martin Luther King Jr.

Connectedness is another fundamental quality that makes nurses great because it enables them to establish relationships with the patients by integrating essential aspects such as trust, respect, and confidentiality. Connectedness refers to the individual and meaningful relationships that the nurses develop and share with the patients. Put, it is the symbiotic relationship between the patients and the nurses. In the hospital, the nurses have a responsibility to ensure that the patients feel safe with their knowledge and experience. As the patients develop trust, the nurses should also establish a conscious commitment to care for the patient. Connectedness is vital because it enables the nurses to use a patient-centered approach when developing the relationship and meeting the patient's needs.

The nurses also respect the uniqueness of each of their patients' and strive to understand their response to changes in health, hence allowing them to develop meaningful relationships with the patients. The bonds are essential because sometimes the patients present the needs of the spirit that emanate from deep within the individual. Connectedness is necessary during such conditions because it enables the nurses to meet the spiritual needs of the patients, promotes healing, growth, and comfort to both the patient and the nurse. Lastly, connectedness makes nurses great because it enhances confidentiality between the nurses, patients, and their families. It is essential to ensure that from the standpoint of trust, the patients are assured that their medical information is kept confidential. Confidentiality is not also a paramount foundation in the healthcare profession, and it opens the door for more in-depth introspective conversations whereby the health care professional plays the role of an active listener. The connection is enhanced because the patients become more forthcoming and honest. When the patients feel understood and respected, their experience in the healthcare facility is a positive one.

Chapter 12
Character of Nurse

"Character is like a tree and reputation like a shadow. The Shadow is what we think of it; the tree is the real thing." - Abraham Lincoln

Professionalism encompasses the display characteristics and behaviors associated with a subjective approach towards the effective execution of an assigned position and task. Nearly every profession needs an employee whose personality is kind, but whose vital characteristic, particularly in the field of nursing, is in healthcare.

Conventionally, Nursing is considered to be the 'care profession.' People who study, career nursing have been stereotyped as 'careful,' 'serving' and 'sympathetic,' nevertheless, Nursing is a career that is truly inspiring and deeply rewarding. In health care, observing the mental parameters of a patient can be an important measure of how fast he or she can recover physically. The nursing staff's personality and the quality of care a patient receives can have a significant impact on their mental state. Nurses must exemplify empathy and sympathy towards patients, as these as emblematic attributes required of a successful and great nurse. For this reason, nurses are the cornerstone of healthcare systems, and frequent interaction with patients characterizes their position. They constitute a precious resource, and in healthcare centers, they are generally the first point of contact.

In the character of nurse reveal a few essential things like:

Communication Skills: A great nurse has excellent communication skills, mainly when talking and listening. They can solve problems and interact efficiently with patients and families based on team and patient feedback. Nurses must always be on top of their game and make sure that everyone else understands their patients. A truly stellar nurse can support and anticipate their requirements for their clients.

Attitude: Caring is the core of the profession of nursing. It underlies everything you do, even when your change becomes hectic, in a caring approach.

Excellent listening skills: A good nurse is sympathetic and can listen to their customers and colleagues concerning having sound clinical skills.

Emotional Stability: Nursing is a stressful task where there are prevailing traumatic circumstances. It is essential to be able to recognize pain and death without allowing it to become personal. An excellent nurse is capable of managing the stress of sad circumstances, but also drawing power from the fantastic results that can and do occur.

Empathy: Great nurses have pain and pain, empathy for patients. They can feel compassion and be comfortable. But be ready for the occasional bout of compassion fatigue; it occurs to the most significant nurses. Learn how to acknowledge and cope effectively with the symptoms.

Flexibility: Being flexible and rolling with the punches is a staple of any profession, but for nurses, it is particularly essential. In terms of working hours and duties, an excellent nurse is flexible. Nurses are often needed to work for longer periods of overtime, late or overnight shifts, and weekends, like physicians.

Attention to Detail: Every step in the medical field is one that can have far-reaching consequences. A great nurse pays excellent attention to detail and is careful not to skip steps or make errors. Precision and accuracy are vital towards paying attention to detail.

Interpersonal Skills: Nurses are the link between doctors and patients. A great nurse has excellent interpersonal skills and works well in a variety of situations with different people. They work well with other nurses, doctors, and other members of the staff.

Physical Endurance: Frequent physical activities, long-term standing, lifting heavy items, and performing several daily taxing maneuvers are the staples of nursing life. It certainly isn't a desk job.

Problem Solving Skills: An excellent nurse, as they emerge, can believe rapidly and solve issues. Nurses always need to be on hand to fix a problematic scenario with sick patients, trauma cases, and emergencies. Whether it's family handling, treating a patient, dealing with a doctor, or managing the employees, having excellent problem-solving abilities are an excellent nurses top quality.

Quick Response: Nurses must be prepared to react to emergencies and other emerging circumstances rapidly. Healthcare work is quite often merely the answer to sudden incidences, and nurses must always be ready for the unexpected. Staying on their feet, maintaining their head cool in a crisis, and being calm in a nurse is excellent characteristics.

Respect: Respect is reciprocal. It's a lengthy way to respect. Great nurses appreciate individuals and regulations. At all times, they stay impartial and are aware of the demands for confidentiality and distinct cultures and traditions. Above all, they respect the patient's desires himself or herself. The hospital employees and each other are recognized by great nurses, understanding that the patient comes first. And nurses are extremely regarded in exchange for respecting others.

Chapter 13
Change Agent

"Change the way you look at things and the things you look at change" – Wayne W. Dwyer

Change is a term that conjures up pictures and emotions of all types for individuals. There is an inextricable link between evolution and health care. In today's setting, health care organizations are always faced with the need to adapt to modifications from many sources like improvements in medical care and technology, raising patients' requirements and expectations that are actively engaged in their health and well-being and changing reimbursement models that emphasize importance rather than quantity.

We said, therefore, that changing for nurses is a fact of life. Nurses are the world's most significant health care workforce. To navigate through change, every nurse must have powerful management abilities with a focus on the patient and providing secure and reliable care. Nursing has a critical contribution to healthcare reform and requests for a healthcare system that is secure, quality, patient-centered, accessible and affordable To deliver these results, all nurses (from the chief nursing officer to the staff nurse) need to understand how the practice of nursing needs to be dramatically different in order to deliver the expected level of quality care and to participate proactively and passionately in the change.

We can play a crucial role in shaping the future health care system. From technology that helps improve our processes and healthcare delivery efficiency to evidence-based practice that develops our care's effectiveness, we need to be responsive to changes. There are transformative changes in healthcare for which nurses are well placed to contribute and lead due to their position, their education, and the respect they have gained. Nurses need to be a significant player in shaping these changes; nurses need to know the factors that drive change, the requirements for change in practice, and the abilities (knowledge, skills, and attitudes) that will be required for wide-ranging achievement in both the personal and system. These modifications will involve a new or improved skillset for wellness and population care, with a renewed focus on patient-centered care, coordination of care, data analysis, and enhancement of quality.

A positive change agent is a coach who uses behaviors such as role modeling, instruction, and facilitation to inspire change for colleagues and nursing leaders. Positive agents for change can provide a forum to influence and support others in the effective execution of programs in healthcare industries. The beneficial change agent that helps your colleagues make a fantastic difference in the health care experience of your patients.

Consider a "shared attitude to leadership" when performing a shift in the unit. Shared governance brings ideas for improving nursing quality from bedside to boardroom, establishing a forum for nurses to select changes that can increase patient results, reduce health care disparities, and advance care delivery. Shared governance also fosters knowledge of how clinical practice and dedication to its achievement will positively affect the shift. As a change agent, the nurse should use his/her behaviors, including guidance, facilitation, and inspiration to inspire others toward change, altering human capabilities, and supporting and influencing others toward change.

Transformation and the necessary modifications will not be straightforward on an individual or system-level basis. Individually, it needs an examination of one's expertise, abilities, and attitudes, and whether that makes you willing to contribute or resist the shift that is to come. At an organizational level, it needs an assessment of the organization's mission, objectives, partnerships, procedures, management, and other vital components and then revision of them, thereby disrupting stuff as we understand them. The truth is that the function of everyone is to change the patients, doctors, nurses, and other healthcare professionals throughout the entire care continuum. Success will be achieved if all healthcare practitioners work together to transform and leverage each provider's contribution to the complete range of practice. It needs inter-professional cooperation to make patient-centered, coordinated care, and it is a chance for nursing to shine.

Some of the obstacles to becoming a significant change leader require an exhibition of education and training to the fullest point. Nurses must also be acknowledged as a fully functioning discipline in the delivery of health care and as a complete partner in decision- making on health care.

Chapter 14
Clarity in Nursing

"A lack of clarity could put the brakes on any journey to success" – Steve Maraboli

According to Val Saintsbury, "Nurses dispense comfort, compassion, and caring without even a prescription."

The role of clarity is to apply the scope of practice to the provision of workplace nursing care. The healthcare profession's value statements emphasize respect, empathy, transparency, and care. The absence of kindness harms patients, especially the elderly and end-illness sufferers. Multiple studies have shown that the compassion level shown by nurses is often affected by variables such as staffing levels, skill mix, and weak dependence.

Together with patients and peers, good nurses are great communicators. Effective communication leads to beneficial results for patients. Nurses elevate spirits and calm nerves as the first point of contact. They can also make sure patients know the directions and expectations of physicians.

A central skill is the capacity to explain complex data naturally. Usually, patients seek clarity, and expressively talking makes it simpler for patients to understand the data. Transparency enables patients to correctly follow instructions, thereby improving the likelihood of beneficial medical results.

To make informed choices, patients must comprehend all hazards, dosages, and complications. Most importantly, nursing employees should endeavor to create patients feel comfortable. Reliable and accountable are competent nurses. They correctly and diligently finish all their duties and show attention to detail. There is little room for error in the patient assessment and treatment process. An error has the potential to endanger the lives of patients. Medical personnel should develop management abilities; the profession needs professionals. This allows employees to deal with the nature of their duties. Working long hours, including weekends and holidays, is prevalent for nurses.

In this sector, patience is the leading quality. It enables even under pressure experts to remain calm. Also, when dealing with angry patients or peers, nurses are taught to prevent confrontation. Staying calm is a sure-fire way to deal professionally with distressing circumstances.

For people who care about people, including the elderly and kids, the profession can be gratifying. Providing emotional support and encouragement make it possible for patients to feel uplifted and remain positive.

Infrastructure for health care and inefficient job procedures can lead to stress on nursing employees. This, in turn, decreases the amount of time invested in the immediate patient care drastically. Also known to cause nurse burnout are these factors, which can lead to lousy recruitment and retention of skilled personnel.

Lower nurse-patient ratios on another level can translate into a rise in mortality. This shows that in terms of patient safety, nurse staffing, and clinical effectiveness play a crucial role. Meanwhile, the innovative design of healthcare facilities and optimized job procedures assist in enhancing recruitment and retention of employees. Therefore, clarity is an essential feature of nursing.

Chapter 15
Customer Service

"There are no traffic jams along the extra mile" – Roger Staubach

Customer service in health care is the delivery that provides support and care for their customers. The patients, their families, and the communities that are served are the customers. Every day, millions of individuals have access to health care services. Whether emergency care, regular examinations, laboratory examination, radiology, surgery, etc., Healthcare is one of the world's most extensive services, affecting millions across the globe. The healthcare system is set up to enable patients to choose their supplier and choose where to receive care.

The client support service is vital for the health care industry. There is no doubt that a team of skilled customer support managers not only acts as a bridge between patients and hospitals but also improves therapy efficacy while coordinating the same. The customer service is depending on the management staff, nurses, and doctors. When we talk about the role of the nurse in healthcare is most important.

For hospitals, doctors' offices, and other medical outlets, nurses play a significant customer service role. Nurses are the ones with the most common, direct communication between patients. They function as liaisons and leave enduring impressions between doctors and patients. It will improve customer satisfaction by providing outstanding customer service to patients. A few essential things every nurse must be aware of while dealing clients are as follows:

Rapport with clients:

The customer service team should maintain a close rapport with every patient. Once a satisfied patient goes home after getting cured in a quick time, then definitely it creates a favorable image in the mind of the patients.

Courtesy and Respect:

Always respect your patient. Ethical behavior at the reception or over a telephone from a customer care executive instantly touches the heart of the patients.

Connect with clients and be personable:

Listen to them carefully. Use touch when appropriate, make eye contact, and do not rush interactions with patients. Acknowledge that you understand the patients' desires and concerns by summarizing and stating them back to the patient and verifying.

Stay informed:

Addressing patients does not only mean keeping close watch solely on their bills and records, but it only implies that the customer care employees should resolve the patient's doubts.

Use appropriate language:

To discuss medical information and communicate using language that is easily understood by the client. Using overly-sophisticated medical terminology may cause unnecessary confusion and sometimes patient anxiety when delivering information concerning a medical diagnosis.

Good manners are going to get you anywhere: Civility and good manners are a part of trust and expertise. Do not conceal the reality, even if it causes you problems. Treat patients as you would like to be treated. Speaking the right words can show respect.

Don't dispute, argue, or match wits:

It's rude to tell patients they're incorrect about anything. They should still be respected, even if they have inaccurate data. If you disagree with them, clarify politely why they are not necessarily right in their point of perspective. Your objective should be explained and communicating and then demonstrating and communicating. Help patients know what happens when they receive therapy. In the system of things, patients should feel that they are just as crucial as you are.

Use simple and easy to understand explanations:

Throwing around complicated jargon may be enjoyable, but it leads to misunderstandings and mistakes at times. No one wants errors in the healthcare setting of today. Always be careful not to cloud your explanations with excessive and complex repetition. Conciseness is very key. In natural, declarative phrases, real experts convey information in the easiest way possible.

Quick response and being alert:

Patients want immediate attention from hospital staff. So, responsiveness is critical if a health care center wishes to win against its competitors. Being responsive means attending to their queries instantly and as well as supplying the necessary medicines and tablets straight to the house of the patients if they need the same urgently.

Frequently thank your client:

The healthcare sector is all about patients. Their belief and faith will multiply the number of future patients in your hospital. So, it is imperative for the customer service team to thanks each patient from time to time to make them feel special.

Chapter 16
Charismatic

"Charisma is the transference of enthusiasm" – Ralph Archbold

Charismatic is concerned with exceptional communication skills, the ability to keep in close contact with others, encouraging others to join in. Charismatic leaders have qualities that are difficult to pin down, but that attracts supporters and inspire individuals to act. Transformational leaders are often extremely charismatic because they can initiate and maintain an exceptional level of organizational change.

According to Weber, in 1947 described the charisma as a unique personality characteristic that gives a person 'superhuman' or exceptional powers and is reserved for a few, is of divine origin, and results in the person being treated as a leader.

Charismatic leaders also show particular kinds of behaviour, as they are powerful models of convictions and values that their followers want to embrace, seem competent to their supporters, clear ideological goals with moral overtones, communicate elevates expectations to followers, and show trust in the ability of followers to satisfy these expectations. The effect of this conduct is to enhance the feeling of competence and self-efficacy of followers, which in turn improves their efficiency, prompting task-relevant motives in followers that may include affiliation, authority, or appreciation. Leaders of hospitals and health care systems need to be critical thinkers, creative problem-solvers, and efficient in prioritizing goals. Contemporary healthcare environments are defined by discontinuous change, enhanced expectations of all service users, increased professional accountability and political pressure for effectiveness, integrating standardized, readily measurable results, technologically driven change, aging population, and enhanced concentrate on the role of management and leadership in clinical practice.

Transformational leadership in nursing highly dependent on charisma, almost to the exclusion of other transformative aspects, and the absence of guidance on how to combine transformative and transactional leadership behavioral characteristics to obtain optimal impact. It's a management quality that can empower employees and facilitate co-operation, creativity, and innovation in nursing.

The following are some of the most prominent characteristics of charismatic leadership in nursing.

Charismatic leaders have extraordinary skills in communication. This helps to motivate employees through tough times and also helps them stay grounded when things are good.

Though they have a compelling personality, a charismatic leader also has maturity and character.

Charismatic leaders also have a sense of humility. They place a lot of value on each employee and have the ability to listen to their concerns truly.

Successful charismatic leaders are also compassionate. Charisma can exist without substance, but only for a short time.

Charismatic leaders are genuinely confident. They are the glass half full kind of people and are comfortable with who they are.

One of the first things that you'd notice about a charismatic leader is their warm, open, and positive body language. They make eye contact with were that they are talking to, smile, and introduce themselves to strangers with the genuine joy of building a new connection.

Charismatic leaders are excellent listeners. When they listen to you, they don't fidget or look distracted.

A charismatic leader understands that he has certain qualities that make him different from others and that these are the qualities that get his attention and make him charismatic.

According to Davidhizar R, 1993, charismatic leadership can positive influences of charisma in transformational leadership are identified as follows:

Self-esteem:

Having a positive self-regard is an essential personal characteristic of leadership, which is projected onto followers. Charismatic leaders are confident, highly enthusiastic, and have a high sense of self-worth. These characteristics are essential determinants of influence as subordinates (followers) are unlikely to follow a leader who appears lacking in self-confidence, personal ability, or has little understanding of organizational goals and the broader environmental influences.

Focus on People:

Within the nursing profession, the ability to relate to other members of the team who are likely to possess high levels of interpersonal skills themselves is an essential determinant of active leadership/ influence. This is especially important given that the ability to sustain and develop human relationship is an integral component of effective practice. The charismatic/transformational nursing leader ensures that relationships with colleagues are used to foster participation in problem-solving and decision-making as a basis for sustaining a commitment to shared goals. Focus on people is one characteristic of charismatic leadership. In other words, the leader who utilizes a charismatic approach is orientated to people and visibly focuses on the human needs of followers. When subordinates present concern, the leader conducts an assessment to find the basis for care."

Vision:

Having an idea is an essential component of leadership for a leader who seeks to lead with charisma. Having a vision for the development of practice, the ward/dept, organization, patient/clients, and other stakeholders involves "knowing where the department, unit or organization is heading and how society will be served." A vision allows followers to reflect on the current state, identify its shortcomings, and become committed to a desirable future state, which is attainable and predicated on known professional/ideological values.

Management of Trust:

It is essential as leaders cannot empower with trust, and trust is critical in the transformational process. Trust is communicated to followers in many different ways, but one of the most important is through leadershipvisibility.

Management of Self:

Confidence that exceptional leaders gain through learning about themselves; their skills, prejudices, talents and shortcomings, self-confidence develops as build on strengths and overcome weaknesses."

Chapter 17
Coachable

"You must always be the apprentice. Even when you become the master" – Christopher Cumby

Coaching is a cooperative relationship between a trained facilitator (coach) and a prepared individual (customer). It is time-limited and concentrated and utilized discussion to assist customers (people or organizations) in attaining their objectives.

Coaching is a relationship of collaboration between a coach and the client, a ready person. It is time-limited and concentrated and utilizes discussions to assist customers in reaching their objectives. It requires the coach's ability to facilitate meaningful conversations and "guide" the customer. Learning begins when the discussion of coaching begins, and new behavior and new procedures are always the final phases of an excellent analysis of coaching. Coaching is not providing guidance, not teaching, and not directing it is a partnership in which the trainer operates like a midwife: supporting, promoting, and assisting the customer through the experience while recognizing the customer as the "making it happen" specialist and individual. To facilitate these coaching conversations, a coach must have the ability to listen, discuss and question; to clarify core values, beliefs, and a sense of purpose; to identify gaps between a client's vision and reality; and to encourage, motivate and instill confidence.

For leaders, executives, teachers, scientists, and professional coaching is the main competency. Coaching enables nurses to participate in discussions and interactions aimed at improving professional development, commitment to the profession, and practice. Individuals behave as trainers or are trained to advance their career and exercise possibilities. They may also use coaching to assist them in making their present roles more enjoyable and satisfied. Besides trends in coaching techniques, there are also untapped possibilities for distinct coaching application fields. Peer, health and interprofessional coaching and succession planning are four fields with excellent potential in nursing. Let's look at each one more closely.

Health Coaching:

Health coaching is a helpful approach to assist nurses in attaining their objectives. Increasingly, patients want to take charge of their health futures, and health coaching allows nurses to use a centered form of communication to deliver patient-centered care. There are currently restricted instances of nurses in literature health coaching. Still, the strategy appears to be a natural fit for the connection between nurse and client where customers articulate their requirements, and the nurse coach asks questions that will assist the client move forward. Coaching customers and patients is another application promising to expand the practice of nursing.

Peer Coaching:

It is possible to use peer coaching to assist nurses in progressing their careers and boosting their job satisfaction. Organizations continue to look for ways to maintain senior nurses and provide possibilities for junior nurses and provide all nurses with practical assistance and support. One way an employer can acknowledge that a nurse's knowledge and dedication and assist other nurses is to provide possibilities for a nurse coach to help a colleague was working on a clinical or professional problem. Peer coaching can also be used to allow employees to talk about their professions and career opportunities.

Recruits or starting professionals within the organization are precious yet fragile resources and need special attention as such. Peer coaching can improve retention by giving fresh workers the abilities and expertise they need to navigate the organization and effectively negotiate with their peers.

Inter-professional Coaching:

The emphasis on promoting inter-professional training and exercise is growing. The ultimate objective is to work in teams to provide extensive care to nurses, physicians, and other healthcare professionals. The emphasis on promoting inter-professional training and exercise is growing. The ultimate objective is to work in teams to provide extensive care to nurses, physicians, and other healthcareprofessionals.

Succession Planning:

Succession scheduling programs for leadership are becoming a primary element of the long- term human resources policies of many organizations. These programs usually include individual and group coaching, mentoring, and internship/job sharing. Coaching is used to determine individual career ambitions, clarify objectives for learning and personaldevelopment, and promote fresh transition leaders.

There are various phases in our careers when looking for possibilities for enrichment. Informal coaching roles are components of their daily operations for many nurses, whether speaking to peers about their career visions or speaking to customers about their health visions. Having a coaching discussion with either a colleague or client is a chance to listen to what might stop them from realizing their ideas. If you are interested in coaching, consider participating in a coach training program that will not only enhance your abilities but also expand your career opportunities.

Chapter 18
Collaborative in Nursing

"Collaboration allows us to know more than we are capable of knowing by ourselves." – Paul Solarz

Collaboration is essential to the practice of nursing and more than communication. Collaboration is a complex, multi-attribute idea. It is described in a multitude of respects, many of which refer explicitly to interdisciplinary cooperation. Attributes recognized by several nursing writers include sharing planning, decision-making, problem-solving, setting objectives, assuming accountability, collaborating, communicating, and publicly coordination. Related ideas are often used as replacements, such as collaboration, joint exercise, and collegiality.

Collaboration is both a process and an outcome in which key stakeholders address shared interest or conflict that cannot be resolved by any person. Any party directly affected by other actions to solve a complicated issue is the main stakeholder. To better comprehend complicated issues, the cooperative method includes a synthesis of distinct views. A collaborative result is the creation of integrative alternatives that go beyond an individual vision to a productive resolution that no single person or organization has been able to achieve.

As a nurse or midwife, for an excellent collaborative relationship, you must have these traits:

Acceptance:

If you're working well on a team, you need to be comfortable with diversity and accept it. Everyone you work with is doubtful to share your race, ethnicity, political opinions, religion, and cultural preferences. Recognizing a difference amongst backgrounds and views can help your team create fresh thoughts and prevent individualistic and one-dimensional approaches, inherently facilitating collaboration for effective results.

Self Awareness:

Do you understand the strengths and weaknesses of your own? You're supposed to. You can maximize your usefulness for the team if you know what you are good at and where you are struggling. Furthermore, create an attempt to comprehend your prejudices. If you have ingrained attractions or aversions to certain concepts, therapies, or patient care techniques, make sure that you understand where those attractions/aversions come from and are willing to protect or reconsider your positions if other people on the team feel differently.

Kindness:

Nobody is perfect, and nobody always agrees with everyone. To work together, you must recognize that individuals are going to create errors, and disputes are going to occur. The right way to deal with a mistake is to assist correct the error and to help ensure that comparable mistakes will not happen in the future. Disagreement can be productive in the event of a dispute, but only if you treat conflict as a chance to improve the team and the work. An intelligent compromise can be the best way forward in many cases.

Patience:

Collaboration requires agreement, and it requires time for a deal. It is essential to stay patient, even in an urgent medical matter and to allow the cooperation to come together. Getting annoyed can generate unhelpful disputes or lead others to withhold their thoughts, which could result in your team missing a prospective diagnosis, therapy option, or solution to the problem.

Flexibility:

An excellent idea/realization can appear at any time in productive cooperation. In fast-moving medical scenarios, this is particularly true. You need to be prepared and willing to adjust on the fly for your team to succeed. That doesn't mean you shouldn't talk if you think an idea is terrible, but it does mean you shouldn't stick out of stubbornness to a previous idea/plan.

Being able to collaborate is just one of the many skills you need to go far in your nursing career.

Chapter 19
Community health in Nursing

"Health equity is everybody's work" – Dr. Anneta Arno

Community health nursing is a discipline that includes evidence-based studies along with developments in science and fresh approaches to health improvement. Practice takes into account the cultural and socio-economic backgrounds of the community's individuals to guarantee suitable communication and sensitivity in working with them.

Community health nurses interact with individuals from various cultural backgrounds, including (but not limited to) those who are disadvantaged and marginalized. In a particular place, a community is a group of individuals that contains areas where individuals reside, work, and go to school. Most individuals are members of various societies. Community health nursing is frequently practiced in places such as towns and rural regions.

Community health nursing is aimed at promoting, protecting, and preserving public health. These fundamental ideas are included in Community health nursing:

- Encourage a healthy lifestyle

- Prevent disease and issues with health

- Provide care directly

- Educate the community on chronic condition management and making the right decisions

- Assess the delivery of patient care and wellness projects of a community Institute program for health and wellness

- The research aimed at improving health care

A nurse who is considering working in community health must be able to assume accountability, act in emergencies, and have practical communication skills. Such nurses must be able to operate independently and collaboratively, maintain patience and discretion in offering health care, and be open to working in both a clinical environment and off-site, such as conducting home visits.

Community health nurses provide an interpretative bridge between the acute industry and services to the community. To advocate and offer a voice to the society, accessing care, they adopt a social model of health. Nurses in community health can simplify health systems, referral pathways, and access to care in a scheme that is often complicated and difficult to navigate.

Community-based health nurses operate in an interdisciplinary team that may include, but are not restricted to, mental health nurses, podiatrists, general practitioners, psychologists, female health nurses, Aboriginal health employees, allied health and hospital facilities.

Community health nurses are appreciated in many environments, including community health clinics, churches, homeless shelters, and schools, for their adaptability and readiness to provide care. These nurses offer patients within their homes with extensive care, at organized events such as health fairs, and art organizations and organizations that serve individuals with specific health requirements. Excellent community practice staff enhances access to care and reduced expenses in university and primary and secondary school nurse-managed clinics. They create and execute corporate wellness programs to support the team and their organizations ' health and productivity.

Community health nurses operate with a variety of partners and suppliers to tackle complicated community problems. This is nowhere more apparent than in present attempts to recognize, reach, and treat individuals living with HIV and AIDS and to assist the elderly handle their chronic health issues efficiently and stay at home. Community or government health nurses may specialize in residential care, case management, clinical, college, or commercial nursing or drug companies' sales. In higher education and clinical research, community health nurses with advanced degrees can also discover the possibilities. The abilities required or these varied fields may differ, but at least nurses should have the degree and sound clinical experience of a bachelor. Nurses who choose traditional public health or home care should understand health problem broadly and are comfortable with independence, change, and uncertainty.

Nurses entering this specialty must emphasize their clinical abilities as well as their critical thinking, advocacy, and analytical abilities. Communities are dynamic, and nurses need to adapt to provide whatever care they need for patients.

Chapter 20
Candor in Nursing

"There is no diplomacy like Candor" – E.V. Lucas

Healthcare professionals must be open and honest with clients when something is wrong within the course of treatment or when there is a tendency for damage or distress. This implies that health care practitioners must inform the client (or, if necessary, the advocate, caregiver, or family of the client) about any information needed while maintaining due healthcare protocol. When something has gone wrong and the patient (or, if necessary, the advocate, caregiver or family of the patient) must be informed, an apology must be made while offering an appropriate solution or help to correct matters (if necessary) fully describe to the patient (or, the advocate, caregiver or family) the brief and long-term impacts of what has occurred.

Healthcare professionals also need to be open and honest with their peers, employers, and appropriate organizations and, when required, participate in reviews and inquiries. It is essential to be open and honest in conversations with regulators/ administrators, respectfully raising issues where necessary.

In nursing or health care professions, the candor focuses not only on the responsibility to be open and honest with patients but also on the need to be open and honest in reporting harmful occurrences or near misses within organizations. A lot of ethical concentrations or values described how a nurse would maintain his or her sincerity in duty; we will talk between a few of them:

All healthcare practitioners have a candor duty a professional obligation when things go wrong to be sincere with patients.

Patients need to be fully informed of their care. You need to discuss the risks as well as the benefits of the options when talking about care options with patients.

A suitable individual must provide the patient with clear, precise data about the hazards associated with the suggested therapy or care and the risks associated with any reasonable alternatives and verify that the patient knows them. You should address the hazard that often happens, severe dangers, although very unlikely, and risks that the patient is likely to believe are essential.

This guidance is not designed for situations where, owing to the natural progression of their disease, the condition of a patient becomes worse. It applies when something goes wrong with a patient's care, and they suffer harm or distress as a result. This guidance also applies in situations where a patient may yet suffer damage or pain as a result of something going wrong with their care.

As a nurse or midwife, you have to talk to the patient as quickly as you realize that something with their care has gone wrong. When you speak to them, they should be supported by someone (for instance, a friend, relative, or professional partner).

It is you're your responsibility to share everything you understand and think to be accurate about what went wrong and why, and what is likely to be the effects. If anything is still unsure, you should clarify and answer any questions honestly. The client should be excused.

Usually, patients want to learn more about what went wrong. But you should offer them the choice that not every detail should be provided. You should try to find out why, if the patient doesn't want more data. If they don't modify their minds after discussion, you should respect their desires as much as possible, * having described the potential implications.

To apologize to a patient does not imply that you accept legal responsibility for what has occurred.

When we apologize to patients and explain what happened, we don't expect you to be responsible for something wrong that wasn't your fault.

We don't want to encourage a formal strategy to apologize as an apology is only valuable if it is real.

Chapter 21
Creativity in Nursing

"You can't use up creativity. The more you use, the more you have" – Maya Angelou

Creativity is an exceptional capacity that creates unexpected yet relevant thoughts and procedures. It is an essential ability for nurse teachers as it allows them to enhance their problem-solving skills, enhance their teaching, improvise teaching and learning strategies, and enhance learning for the participant.

Nursing is as much an art as it is a science (translation: creative art). There are so many items that nurses are already using that have not been invented yet. Cardboard-like funnels, garbage can be used as a tray for medicine, etc. Nurses around the world engage in innovative operations daily, activities that are driven by the need to enhance care results, and decrease health system expenses.

As the complexity of nursing and health care escalates, nurses are asked to give innovative nursing practice alternatives. Dealing with patients of various ages, health circumstances, and backgrounds have made creativity a key element in nursing responsibilities. Nurses that incorporate creativity in inpatient care can decrease health care system expenses and promote developments in the nursing/healthcare sector. Creativity could also be seen as a channel for bridging the gap between theory and practice of nursing. This capability should be embraced by educators and steps taken to improve it over time. The practical approaches mentioned in this paper can assist teachers in strengthening their creativity.

Creativity promotes collaboration and higher satisfaction of patients:

Creativity significantly enhances the partnership and comfort of patients. When the nurse has to cope with uncooperative children on several occasions, creativity will offer her a benefit. A nurse may use toys to improve collaboration when providing care for a child patient. This will also result in increased adherence to drug regimens and changes in dressing. The nurse may also use handcrafts to convey her burning desire to the patient before discharge.

Creativity allows patient care modifications:

It is possible to adapt creativity to nursing procedures and to change the way patient care is transmitted. A stretcher fitted with a cassette for taking X-rays, for example, is an excellent innovation, particularly for various trauma patients. This makes it easy for the employees and their patients to transfer the patient from the stretcher to the radiology bed.

Creativity increases the self-confidence and respect of nurses:

It will assist the nurse in attaining self-belief and happiness by consistently expressing creative thoughts in a working unit. She will realize from day to day that the fun aspects of the job are to discover innovations and ideas. In nursing, creativity should be a key component. A nurse who integrates creativity and innovation will find that it operates as self-empowerment despite direct nursing procedures. The nurse would serve the best possible quality of care with empowerment and enhance the results.

Conclusion

In summary, great nurses were not born with the qualities that made them great, and it takes the acquisition of necessary skills, an exhibition of exemplary behavior such as dogged determination to be the best version of oneself. All 21 C's are the pioneering values that govern who successful nurses are. They are the guiding principles towards maximizing a positive impact in their field and the world around them, leaving legacies that will last lifetimes, and inspiring those looking to be nurses as well. These qualities must be embraced in health care because they ensure the optimal development of patients. All the C's are important, and they should not be viewed in isolation because they are all interconnected in one or more ways to emphasize eloquent and efficient methods by which delivery of quality care and the success of the health care organizations are optimized. Nurses are the backbone of patient service and care. Hence, if nurses engage in self-investment and self-development, they will revolutionize the healthcare industry one day at a time. Nurses are the heart and soul of healthcare and many times are referred to as the healthcare heroes of today and tomorrow. If you are a nurse reading this book, let me take the time to say congratulations on changing and touching lives everyday.